ONE

UNDERSTANDING YOUR DUAL DISEASES

What Is PTSD?

PTSD refers to a set of symptoms and problems that can develop after a traumatic event which is so intensely frightening, dangerous, and uncontrollable that it overwhelms our ability to cope and severely threatens our basic safety. PTSD has many causes.

The trauma might involve surviving a war experience; being a victim of robbery or assault; suffering severe deprivation, such as chronic poverty or starvation; experiencing or observing a violent accident; being physically or sexually abused; growing up with an alcoholic and/or mentally ill parent who said one thing and did another; or some other intense experience that caused feelings of extreme threat and insecurity. Many people ask, "Am I crazy because I have PTSD?" No! PTSD refers to a normal response to an abnormal (traumatic) situation.

The symptoms may show up only during a particular situation and be limited in time. Or they may occur over a long period of time and in a more general way. Consider the case of Mary, who suffered severe symptoms of PTSD. She had been sexually and physically abused by her stepfather from ages three through nine. Because of the intensity of her trauma and the age at which she experienced it, Mary had many symptoms of PTSD. (The clinical names of Mary's symptoms are given in parentheses.)

Mary had almost no memories of her childhood; she had almost no memories of the abuse she experienced (amnesia and dissociation). She had always felt different from others, as if she never fit in (estrangement).

She had always felt that she was the target of others' criticism and that nothing she did was ever good enough (victim-stance thinking and a pessimistic worldview). Mary felt anxious and depressed all the time, and although she pretended to feel things, she had few positive emotions (emotional numbing). Even when she married, Mary did not feel sexually comfortable with her husband and could have sex only after several glasses of wine (trauma-related fears). She had few friends because she could never seem to let anyone get emotionally close to her (fear of abandonment, lack of trust, social isolation). Mary had a problem with her temper and sometimes exploded for trivial reasons (intense anger/rage). At other times she would burst into fears for no apparent reason (flooding). Over time she drank more and more, and felt panicky at the thought of being unable to have a drink. One day Mary saw a television show about childhood abuse (a trigger). Suddenly memories of abuse filled her head, some so vivid she really felt as if she were "back there" (flashback). She was filled with fear, shame, and anger (flooding). Mary called a close friend, who encouraged her to call a therapist and seek help. Mary located a therapist who specialized in PTSD and addiction. With time and hard work, Mary was able to get and stay sober as well as learn to see herself not as a victim, but as a survivor in dual recovery.

The symptoms of PTSD fall into four clusters: *avoidance, reenactments, victim-stance thinking,* and *shame.*

Avoidance

- amnesia (forgetting)

- dissociation ("trancing out"; mentally going away to avoid a painful situation)

- hypervigilance (being overly alert in scanning our surroundings)

- emotional numbing (trying to block feelings to avoid pain)

- controlling behavior (trying to be in charge to regain a sense of power)

- estrangement, or social isolation

Co-occurring Disorders Series

UNDERSTANDING POST-TRAUMATIC STRESS DISORDER AND ADDICTION

Revised

Katie Evans, Ph.D.

HAZELDEN

FORMERLY THE DUAL DIAGNOSIS SERIES

Hazelden
Center City, Minnesota 55012-0176

1-800-328-9000
1-651-213-4590 (Fax)
www.hazelden.org

To request permission, write to
Permissions Coordinator, Hazelden, P.O. Box 176, Center City, MN 55012-0176.
To purchase additional copies of this publication, call
1-800-328-9000 or 1-651-213-4000.

ISBN 13: 978-1-59285-026-6

Editor's note
This material was written to educate individuals about chemical dependency and mental illness. It is not intended as a substitute for professional
medical or psychiatric care.

Any stories or case studies that may be used in this material are compos-
ites of many individuals. Names and details have been changed to protect
identities.

Cover design by Lightbourne
Interior design by Lightbourne

CONTENTS

INTRODUCTION

This workbook is based on professional experience working with individuals who suffer from both post-traumatic stress disorder (PTSD) and addiction. The author is a certified alcohol and drug counselor and has a Ph.D. in clinical psychology. Many people who try to work a program of recovery from addiction have not sought treatment for their survivor issues. Unfortunately, these individuals experience such intense emotional pain that they often see no other course but to resume using mood-altering chemicals. Many give up on recovery because of continued emotional pain or frequent relapse to chemical use. Others spend years in psychotherapy trying to work through the pain of their trauma, while continuing to use chemicals. While others manage to stay sober, they are angry, depressed, and have difficulty in close relationships. This can make them doubt that recovery really "works" for them.

For those who suffer from both PTSD and addiction, an *integrated* recovery program is most helpful because it addresses both at the same time. It focuses on issues and offers suggestions and interventions that are common to both disorders. An integrated approach emphasizes laying a *foundation of safety* before doing emotionally charged work. Working with traumatic memories is not a goal of early dual recovery.

This workbook is based on personal experience as well. The author is working a dual recovery program for both PTSD and addiction. (She was raped as a teen and is the child of two alcoholic parents.) In this workbook, recovery is dealt with not just from the outside but also from the inside.

This workbook gives you (a) an overview of the symptoms and problems associated with PTSD and addiction, (b) a discussion of the dual recovery process, and (c) some helpful tools for the addicted survivor of trauma working on recovery. The workbook is most useful when combined with participation in a Twelve Step program and professional counseling. It should not be considered a substitute for these crucial components of recovery.

Reenactments

- flashbacks of the traumatic event

- nightmares of the event

- flooding (being overwhelmed by feelings or memories)

- overreacting to situations that resemble the event or reacting in self-defeating ways

Victim-Stance Thinking

- distrust of others

- feelings of abandonment

- feelings of helplessness

- great fear of change

- blaming others for our own problems

- unable to take responsibility for own healing process

Shame

- feeling guilty

- feeling as if we are bad or immoral

- feeling as if we are crazy or sick

- feeling as if we are unworthy or are "impostors"

- feeling hopeless and lost on the recovery path

Three factors influence how severe the PTSD will be. *The severity of the trauma* is one factor. Examples of severe trauma include military combat, a catastrophic accident, domestic violence, or sexual abuse. *The age at which the trauma occurs* is another factor: the younger the person, the more severe the symptoms. The third factor is *the degree of support that the victim receives from others during and after the trauma.* This plays a big part in how well the person survives the experience. Being silenced, blamed, and shunned by others revictimizes survivors. This can set up two interlinked themes: "I am not safe" and "No one will help." These survivors are often stuck in both the pain of what was done to them (the trauma) and the lack of support from others (abandonment).

Symptoms of Chemical Dependency

Chemical dependency is a chronic, progressive, and potentially fatal disease. Some symptoms of addiction are *negative consequences* from the use of chemicals and *loss of control* of chemical use. Liver disease, heart disease, or lung cancer are examples of some of the physical problems that addicts may develop. They may experience social problems, such as being fired from a job, fighting with a spouse, or being charged with drunk driving. They may have tried to cut down or stop but failed. Some common symptoms of addiction include

- lying about chemical use, denying or minimizing problems caused by the use of alcohol and other drugs

- preoccupation with use

- failed efforts to cut back, quit, or follow personal rules—such as drinking only with friends or drinking only wine or beer (loss of control)

- increasing frequency, amounts of use, or escalating problems as a result of drinking or using (progression)

- needing more of the chemical to get the same effect (tolerance)

- rapid intake

- protecting the supply/hiding extra "just in case"

- blackouts

- family, work, and legal problems

- withdrawal symptoms, such as the "shakes," restlessness, irritable feelings, or mood swings

- using to avoid withdrawal

Synergism: 1+1=3

Suffering from both PTSD and addiction is *synergistic;* that is, the combined impact on the addicted survivor is greater than the impact of each disease individually. In addition to the symptoms listed above, addicted survivors also experience strong, ongoing feelings of anxiety and depression. So, 1 (PTSD) + 2 (PTSD + addiction) = 3.

Take the example of Mark, a Vietnam veteran. Mark tried psychotherapy once or twice to try to help him with flashbacks of the war, but found that he only "felt worse when he talked about the war." A counselor suggested to Mark that he was an alcoholic, pointing out, for example, that he drank a six-pack a night and that his wife was threatening to divorce him if he didn't stop drinking so much. Bothered by these two problems, and yet too overwhelmed to do anything different, Mark continued to drink. Over a period of time, his mood worsened and he drank even more. Overwhelmed by the memories of his combat experience, Mark tried on several occasions to kill himself while under the influence of alcohol.

Survivors are at high risk for addiction. We often turn to chemicals to "medicate" our pain and begin to believe that *only* chemicals can relieve it. This belief may linger in recovery. It needs to be challenged and then changed, by self-examination and by learning new ways to deal with the pain. Otherwise, we relapse into chemical use.

Newly sober survivors may feel as though their PTSD symptoms are worsening. The chemicals may have helped block painful feelings, which are now returning. Addicted survivors often find themselves in a vicious circle: their chemical use, once a solution, is now part of the problem. Their PTSD fuels their addiction and their addiction fuels their PTSD.

Knowing the symptoms of your illness is an important step in the dual recovery process. The following exercise will help you identify past and present symptoms of both diseases.

It's a good idea to share your responses to this exercise (and to the rest of the exercises in this workbook) with a person you trust, such as a good friend, a Twelve Step sponsor, or a therapist. Sharing is likely to help you keep a balanced, realistic view, and it will give you a source of support and validation.

Recovery Activity: Identifying Symptoms of My Dual Diseases

1. Chemicals helped me block the following unpleasant feelings:

_____

_____

_____

_____

_____

2. My chemical use has caused me several problems, including the following:

_____

_____

_____

_____

_____

3. Two ways that show me my chemical use got out of control:

a. _____

_____

b. _____

4. I believe that I am an alcoholic and/or addict because I exhibit these symptoms of that disease:

5. My PTSD is a result of

6. Others failed to support, protect, or help me deal with my trauma when they

7. My avoidance symptoms of PTSD (see page 4) include the following:

8. My reenactment symptoms of PTSD (see page 5) include the following:

_____

_____

_____

9. I fall into a victim stance (see page 5) when I

_____

_____

_____

10. I feel intense shame (see page 5) when I

_____

_____

_____

11. I believe I suffer from PTSD because I exhibit these symptoms:

_____

_____

_____

_____

12. Two ways my two diseases make each other worse:

a. _____

_____

b. _____

_____

_____

13. I start to think that I will never be able to cope with the pain without chemicals when

_____

_____

_____

14. I finally decided to get help for my problems because

_____

_____

_____

_____

_____

15. Two things that give me some hope that things can get better:

a. _____

_____

_____

b. _____

_____

_____

As you finish this exercise, try not to be too discouraged. Instead, read on to discover some solutions to support your recovery from PTSD and addiction.

TWO

THE PROCESS OF DUAL RECOVERY

Recovery is a process, not an event. That is why we, as addicted survivors, talk about ourselves as being "in recovery," not "recovered."

The process of recovery from PTSD and addiction has five stages: *crisis, building, education, integration,* and *maintenance.* Certain tasks must be accomplished in each stage before advancing to the next. If these tasks and goals are achieved, then transition to the next stage of recovery goes smoothly. If the tasks and goals are not met, going to the next stage is futile; we backslide to a previous stage or may even experience a relapse. On the other hand, if we are progressing in recovery, we typically revisit each stage, but each time at a more advanced level, in an upward spiral.

Crisis Stage

When we are in the crisis stage, we often feel unstable or unsafe. Stopping the use of addictive chemicals and/or clearing all addictive chemicals from our bodies is a difficult, but important start. Maybe we are feeling out of control or even suicidal. Perhaps we are about to relapse (or have relapsed). Maybe we are in an unhealthy or abusive relationship. We may fear that the program doesn't work for us.

A crisis is what brings most of us to treatment. Sometimes the crisis is deliberate and therapeutic, such as a family- or work-sponsored intervention (in which family and friends lovingly confront us with the stressful impact of our chemical use or other negative actions so that we will stop drinking or using other drugs and seek help). More often, the crisis is unplanned, frightening, and confusing. Possibly our marriage has ended, or maybe we face charges for drunk driving or assault. Perhaps we receive an angry phone call from our mother, who has never admitted responsibility for failing to protect us from abuse. In some cases, the custody and the safety of our children has led us to a new bottom.

In a crisis, both physical and emotional safety are a concern. Our physical safety could be endangered, for instance, during withdrawal from chemicals, which can be life threatening if not managed by medical personnel. We can also get ourselves into dangerous situations when intoxicated—fighting in bars, driving drunk, or thinking about overdosing, for example. Our living situation may even be unsafe or unhealthy. If a person who lives with us is drinking, using drugs, or threatening to harm us, we must do what we can to get safe.

Being emotionally safe means taking steps to protect ourselves if others—especially those we live with—ridicule, taunt, threaten, or humiliate us. Our spouses may criticize us, call us names, or threaten to beat us if we aren't compliant. We need to learn how to set boundaries and limits for ourselves and find a safer living environment.

Our goal in the crisis stage of recovery is preventing imminent, serious physical and emotional harm. By completing Step One of the Twelve Steps of Alcoholics Anonymous (AA)—admitting we are powerless over alcohol and that our lives have become unmanageable—we can increase our insight into our chemical use and other areas of our lives. Keep in mind that powerlessness does not mean helplessness. Paradoxically, Step One can help us feel empowered to change unsafe behaviors or situations. The following list describes some strategies for staying safe.

- briefly checking into a hospital for safety or for detoxification
- calling the local crisis line or police
- making a contract for safety (a commitment to a friend, sponsor, or therapist not to attempt suicide or to use chemicals)
- moving in with a relative or going to a women's shelter

- calling a friend for help and support

- attending Twelve Step meetings

- reading the Big Book and other AA-approved literature

- taking nonaddictive medication such as antidepressants if prescribed by a medical doctor who is aware of our addiction

Building Stage

The goal of the building stage of recovery is to become better at protecting and nurturing ourselves. Such skills will make our lives safer (and more pleasant). Some of us never had the chance to learn these skills. And some of us already have many of these skills, but we may have difficulty using them when we are very upset.

An important skill to work on is assertiveness. This means learning how to set boundaries and learning to say no.

We need to take every opportunity to practice setting boundaries, both externally and internally. An external boundary is a limit we set in response to someone or something outside ourselves, such as telling a critical parent not to call more than once a week. An internal boundary is saying no to all forms of harmful self-talk—for example, the endless feelings of shame that arise when we feel someone has criticized us.

Other types of assertiveness include expressing our concerns to others directly, asking for help, and negotiating compromises.

We can further protect and nurture ourselves by completing Steps Two and Three. Step Two can enhance our sense of faith and hope, our sense that someone "out there" can help us and that things are better today than yesterday. Step Three can help us learn to let go of the obsessive need to control everything, by turning over control to our Higher Power, thus ridding ourselves of useless fear and worry.

Some additional skills we may find helpful in recovery include

- practicing relaxation and meditation

- creating a schedule that includes a balance of work activities, self-care activities, health and fitness, and time with family and friends

- learning self-defense techniques

- learning to express feelings by sharing in Twelve Step meetings

- practicing complimenting ourselves

- participating in a dual same-sex recovery group

- forgiving ourselves for being human

Education Stage

In the education stage of recovery, the goal is to transform our sense of self from that of victim to survivor and ultimately a thriver. We deepen our understanding of our dual diseases, recognize their impact on our lives, and learn what we can do to promote our own recovery. We seek support from others to understand the causes of, and remedies for, our diseases. We work at acknowledging our suffering and honoring the incredible strength it has taken to survive and enter recovery. We want to begin to feel that we are truly survivors filled with courage, not victims filled with shame. We ultimately become thrivers when we can see the promises in the Big Book come alive in our lives.

We are not responsible for the cause of our diseases, but we are responsible for finding solutions to manage them. If we understand their processes and can name our symptoms and their roots, we can become stronger as we overcome our trauma and learn that we no longer have to be victims or even survivors. We are thrivers!

Reading books, listening to tapes, and attending workshops and lectures about addiction and PTSD are important tactics in the education stage. By attending and participating actively in meetings where other survivors discuss their recovery, we can celebrate the survivors' strengths and learn helpful ways to express and cope with pain. There are Twelve

Step meetings, such as Incest Anonymous (IA) and Adult Children of Alcoholics (ACOA), for survivors of some forms of trauma. Other community-sponsored meetings which are not Twelve Step-focused, but which can still be very powerful and healing, include Adults Molested as Children (AMAC) and various groups for Vietnam veterans.

During this stage of recovery, we need to try to remember that our own recovery comes first. If we are triggered and begin to feel overwhelmed when doing education work, we need to stop and use our safety skills until we feel safe and sober again. We also need to beware of taking on too much of the pain of others, trying to "rescue" others, or starting romances with other survivors when we are early in recovery and possibly vulnerable to exploitation or at least diversion from our recovery. Many of us are nurturers and natural caretakers of others. However, we neglect our own self-care. This needs to change.

Integration Stage

The goal of the integration stage is to be able to safely and fully experience, in the here and now, all of our actions, thoughts, feelings, bodily sensations, and memories. We want to feel comfortable alone and with other people. Step by step and day by day, we walk through the stages of recovery. We will learn to laugh and not take ourselves so seriously.

Trauma occurred because we couldn't successfully fight back or escape the shock that overwhelmed us. And the trauma worsened because we couldn't stop to process our grief and loss and get validation and support from others. Typically, we coped in the only other way left (other than death): we "disconnected" from ourselves and others as a last-ditch solution to an intolerable situation. Alcohol and other drugs helped us unplug from life.

Dissociation refers to our mentally checking out. When we dissociate, we usually develop at least three parts to handle the trauma: (1) the *wounded* part, to carry our pain, fear, and hurt. The wounded part craved alcohol and other drugs to numb the pain; (2) the *protector* part, to help us cope. The protector part may have consumed us as we played it tough and often said, "I don't need anything from anybody"; and (3) the *nurturing* part, to reduce our feelings of abandonment. The nurturing part of us has been underdeveloped. Learning to comfort ourselves is very important.

Dissociation often works so well that it becomes habitual. We may come to rely on it to help us cope with many aspects of our lives. Chemicals reinforce this habit; they, too, disconnect us from ourselves and others and block true awareness.

Unfortunately, this survival strategy has its costs. Apart from the original trauma, we have experienced many additional shocks and losses because of our PTSD and addiction. Perhaps we've run away from home or quit school early to escape an abuser. Perhaps we've lost jobs or marriages because of our addiction. We've lost not only our innocence and faith but also, when we're in recovery, our best "friend" in the world: alcohol and drugs. We have a great deal of unfinished business from the past stored in our wounded part—which keeps our energy for growth unavailable. Our protector part continues to be overly controlling, hostile, critical, or "nice." Our nurturing part either remains underdeveloped or gets short-circuited. And our parts don't work well together because they are dissociated.

We continue our dual recovery by striving to rediscover, reclaim, and reconnect with all of our "parts" so that we can feel like complete human beings. By gradually allowing ourselves to become aware of all our thoughts, actions, and feelings, and by working through them and accepting them, we can put it all together and become integrated. We also need to grieve our losses and let go of the past by working through our anger and depression, by reflecting on and accepting the impact the losses have had on our lives.

Work on integrating can proceed in a number of ways. Continued work on Step Four can be helpful: an accurate inventory of ourselves can enhance our self-esteem. Some other ways to work on integration issues include the following:

- keeping a daily journal to reflect on our experiences

- writing poetry, painting pictures, or using other artistic means to express feelings

- looking at old photographs to help remember the past and processing the feelings that come up

- writing letters to our other parts (wounded, protector, nurturing)

- visiting a place associated with the loss, such as a childhood home or a war memorial

- taking part in healing rituals, such as literally burying a token of the past

- practicing meditation

- going to meetings

- working with others who are in need

As always, we need to keep safe. Integration work can cause pain, and we can go only as far and fast as we can tolerate. Take one day at a time.

The help of a professional who understands dual recovery from PTSD and addiction can be invaluable in this stage. He or she will notice any dissociation and can help with such tools as hypnotherapy. Working with a professional is particularly important if we plan to confront an abuser or if we have severe symptoms of dissociation (hallucinatory-type flashbacks, large memory gaps in both the remote and recent past that are not due to a blackout, and flooding that incapacitates us). It is important to feel safe with this professional. Make sure he or she is are trained in survivor and addiction therapies.

Maintenance Stage

The final stage of recovery is the maintenance stage. Since we are "recovering" and not "recovered," we need to keep our recovery program active and ongoing. We want to keep an ever-vigilant eye toward preventing a relapse to either of our illnesses. We also want to continue to grow more fully as human beings. Working Steps Ten through Twelve and continuing to participate in Twelve Step meetings and psychotherapy sessions are some ways to do this. Service work—whether through being a sponsor in a Twelve Step program or lobbying for laws to help other survivors—can also be an important part of our work in this stage. Having learned new solutions for old problems and transformed our sense of the past, we are free to move forward into the future, one day at a time. The promises of recovery are now coming true.

THREE

EVALUATING YOUR PROGRESS AND NEEDS IN RECOVERY

The next exercise will help you determine your stage of recovery. Together with the information in the preceding sections, this exercise will suggest issues you might address on your own or with the help of friends or professionals.

Recovery Activity:
Your Stage of Recovery—A Self-Evaluation

In the following section, circle the number of each item that applies to you.

Crisis Stage

1. I regularly feel as if my life is out of control and unmanageable.

2. I sometimes feel that death is the only relief I may ever know from my pain.

3. The only way I know to stop the pain is to get drunk or high.

4. I often feel that the program doesn't work for me.

5. I often think about the "good old days" when I used to drink and use drugs.

6. I often question whether I am really an addict and/or alcoholic.

7. Hurting others or myself somehow helps my emotional pain.

8. I often question whether I really have PTSD.

9. I am currently in a living situation or relationship that poses an immediate danger to my health or safety.

10. I am in a living situation or relationship in which I face regular and severe criticism, ridicule, threats, and harassment.

In the following sections, circle the number of each item that does not apply to you.

Building Stage

1. I am usually comfortable calling my sponsor or other supportive person when I am having a problem.

2. I think asking for help is a sign of strength.

3. For the most part, I can tell someone no if I really don't want to do something.

4. I generally stand up for myself.

5. When someone criticizes me, I no longer feel overwhelmed with hurt.

6. I usually find that I can express my needs and opinions without blowing up.

7. Even when I have many things to do, I usually know where to start and what I need to do to get them done.

8. I can usually tell someone directly when he or she has hurt my feelings or made me mad.

9. I rarely engage in sexual activity when I don't want to (even if it means hurting my partner's feelings).

10. For the most part, I find that I can get organized and accomplish what I set out to do.

11. I usually take time to rest and relax and be good to myself.

12. I seldom find myself reacting impulsively or overreacting to situations and people.

13. I know how to manage flooding of my emotions, so I can generally handle painful feelings.

14. For the most part, I can put worries out of my head after I have done what I can.

Education Stage

1. I am generally familiar with the symptoms of both PTSD and addiction, and I understand how they apply to me.

2. I have a pretty good sense of what I need to do to recover from my dual diseases.

3. I have spent some time reading about and/or listening to knowledgeable people talk about the causes and remedies of my addiction and PTSD.

4. I can discuss what my dual recovery issues are and what I need to do to work on them.

5. I have some idea why certain things are triggers for me.

6. I have connected with others who have the same issues that I have.

7. I have shared my story with others and am becoming more comfortable doing this.

8. I generally accept those things I am responsible for and can hold others accountable for what they are responsible for.

9. I can admit my mistakes and apologize to others without feeling ashamed.

10. I know that I am not alone and that I am one of many survivors in recovery.

11. I know that I no longer have to be a victim, that I am a survivor.

12. I know my strengths and usually feel good about myself.

Integration Stage

1. I usually have no trouble staying in the here and now, and I don't "lose" periods of time.

2. I know what I am feeling and why I am feeling that way.

3. I know how to manage my triggers.

4. For the most part, I have eliminated self-defeating behavior from my life.

5. My memories of the past are not vague or particularly overwhelming.

6. Generally, I know who I am and what I believe.

7. I have grieved my losses and have come to accept them.

8. I have stopped feeling stuck on any of my recovery issues.

9. I know my "parts," and they usually work well together.

10. I find that I am usually at peace with myself.

Maintenance Stage

1. I know that I am recovering and will always need to work a program.

2. I routinely take the time for reflection to see how I'm doing in my recovery and to spot potential problems.

3. I continue to find new ways and new situations in which to grow.

4. I still work at deepening my spiritual program.

5. I'm trying to carry the message, even if in just a small way.

If you circled *any* of the items in the crisis section, get help *now* from friends and/or professionals. Also complete the safety plan exercise on page 25.

If you marked two or more items in any of the other stages, you need to work on that stage as well. Always work on the earlier stages first.

No matter what your stage of recovery, it's a good idea to complete the next exercise, "My Safety Plan." If you begin to feel unsafe for any reason, at any time, put this plan into effect. Safety is the foundation for a dual recovery program for PTSD and addiction.

Later exercises address issues relevant to the building, education, and integration stages. This workbook does not include exercises for the crisis stage, other than the safety plan. (But remember, if you are in crisis, seek help *now*.) Also, there are not any specific exercises for the maintenance stage. Instead, a section on relapse prevention has been included.

Recovery Activity: My Safety Plan

1. I feel unsafe (or I want to drink or use) when

_____

_____

_____

2. When I feel unsafe, some safe places I could go include

_____

_____

_____

3. Some people I feel are safe and supportive for my dual recovery include (write down their names and phone numbers here)

_____

_____

_____

4. When I feel unsafe, I can do these three things to stay safe:

a. _____

b. _____

c. _____

5. When I feel like I want to drink or use drugs, I can do these three things to stay sober and safe:

a. _____

b. _____

c. _____

If you begin to feel unsafe for any reason, put this plan into effect.

Recovery Activity: Building My Safety Skills

If we have strong skills to protect and nurture ourselves, we can stay safe. The following exercise can help those of us in the building stage to develop these skills.

1. Read a book or listen to an audiotape on assertiveness and on relaxation. Write down the names of the books or tapes you chose; then list the two most important things you learned from them.

_____

_____

_____

2. Describe a time when you told someone you disagreed with his or her opinion. How and when did you do this? How did you feel? Why was it okay for you to do so?

_____

_____

_____

_____

3. Think of a time you said no to someone, and explain how it felt. Why was it okay to do so?

_____

_____

_____

_____

4. Give an example of a time someone asked you a question you were not comfortable answering, and you stated clearly that you would rather not respond.

_____

_____

_____

_____

5. Name a boundary you set lately that you feel good about.

_____

_____

_____

6. Name a boundary that you need to set but haven't yet. What fear has made you unable to set this boundary? How might you feel less fearful?

_____

_____

_____

7. Why is it important to let go of whether the other person will still like you *before* you set a boundary?

_____

_____

_____

8. Think of a time you have been angry recently but did not express your anger. Describe the situation. Why didn't you express how you felt? What could you do about this? Was the situation safe for you to discuss your anger or resentment?

_____

_____

_____

_____

_____

_____

9. List two healthy ways to express anger.

   a. _____

   _____

   _____

   b. _____

   _____

   _____

10. List two helpful ways to release stress and relax.

    a. _____

    _____

    _____

    b. _____

    _____

    _____

11. List two ways to manage feelings of depression.

    a. _____

    _____

    _____

    b. _____

    _____

    _____

12. Think of a time you asked someone you felt safe with to help you with something. How did you feel? How might you do this again?

    _____

_____

_____

13. It is important to make time for yourself on a regular basis. What can you do for yourself this week? in future weeks? How can you have fun, relax, and take yourself less seriously?

_____

_____

_____

14. Think of something you've wanted to do for a long time. Imagine that your Higher Power is making this happen for you. Develop a step-by-step plan to accomplish this goal and ask for guidance to get around obstacles that might get in the way.

_____

_____

_____

15. Identify three of your strengths.

a. _____

_____

_____

b. _____

_____

_____

c. _____

_____

_____

16. List three things you do that you feel good about.

a. _____

_____

_____

b. _____

_____

_____

c. _____

_____

_____

Recovery Activity:
Education Stage—Emerging from Victim to Survivor

This exercise is for readers working on the education stage.

1. I have learned that I am not a victim. I am a survivor because

a. _____

_____

_____

b. _____

_____

An example of victim-stance thinking is when

_____

_____

_____

I know I give my power away when

_____

_____

_____

The three most important elements of my recovery program for my addiction and trauma issues are

a. _____

_____

b. _____

_____

c. _____

_____

2. I am learning more about my recovery from PTSD and addiction by doing these things:

a. _____

_____

_____

b. _____

_____

_____

I have learned that some of my PTSD symptoms include the following:

_____

_____

_____

Three reasons why staying clean and sober help me in my PTSD recovery program are

a. _____

_____

_____

b. _____

_____

_____

c. _____

_____

_____

3. Attending a support or therapy group regularly is important for
me because

_____

_____

_____

4. What I find most helpful about my support or therapy group is that

_____

_____

_____

5. Sometimes I have found it difficult to tell my story to others because

_____

_____

_____

6. Some things that I could do to make telling my story easier include

_____

_____

_____

7. Thinking of myself as a survivor in recovery, not a victim, helps me by

_____

_____

_____

Recovery Activity: Integration Stage

The two parts of the following exercise, "Learning about the Different Parts of Me" and the "Grief and Loss Inventory," are for readers working on the integration stage. The first will help us get to know our different parts better. The second will help us identify where we are in our grief process. Remember that a trained therapist is needed to help with successful integration.

PART 1: LEARNING ABOUT THE DIFFERENT PARTS OF ME

My Wounded Part

1. My feelings are easily hurt when

_____

_____

2. I feel alone and abandoned when

_____

_____

3. I feel scared and frightened when

_____

_____

4. I get triggered (and may begin to cry uncontrollably) when

_____

_____

5. I feel ashamed when

_____

_____

6. I feel sad and depressed when

_____

_____

7. I feel small, like a little child, when

_____

_____

8. I most likely flood with any or all of these feelings when

_____

_____

9. It's okay to have these feelings, because

_____

_____

10. A helpful way for me to soothe and calm myself when upset is to

_____

_____

My Protector Part

1. I find that I become defensive when

_____

_____

2. I sometimes try to control a situation or person when

_____

_____

3. I find that I blow up easily at other people when

_____

_____

4. I am very critical of myself when

_____

_____

5. I am critical of others when

_____

_____

6. One good thing about protecting myself by being controlling, angry, critical, or "nice" is that

_____

_____

7. One problem about the way I protect myself is that

_____

_____

8. One way I can protect my sobriety is to

_____

_____

My Nurturing Part

1. I seem to have a hard time taking care of myself when

_____

_____

2. One way I can take better care of myself when I am feeling sad or hurt is to

_____

_____

3. I have learned that it is okay to make mistakes because

_____

_____

4. To forgive myself after making a mistake, I will

_____

_____

5. I am taking better care of my physical health by

_____

_____

6. I am taking better care of my mental health by

_____

_____

7. I am taking better care of my spiritual health by

_____

_____

8. An example of how I can take better care of my sobriety is to

_____

_____

9. To improve my self-care, I need to work on

_____

_____

Working as a Team

1. I can soothe my wounded part and protect and nurture myself by

   _____

   _____

2. My protector part can help me nurture myself and reduce the pain of my wounded part by

   _____

   _____

3. Ways my protector part can do this include the following:

   a. _____

   _____

   b. _____

   _____

4. My nurturing part sometimes causes problems for my wounded and protector parts when

   _____

   _____

5. I feel most like a team and most together when

   _____

   _____

6. I could feel this way more often by

_____

_____

Part 2: Grief and Loss Inventory

1. Addiction and trauma cause many losses. I feel the saddest about losing the following:

   a. _____

   _____

   b. _____

   _____

   c. _____

   _____

2. I get angry when I think about how I lost the following:

_____

_____

3. I feel hurt when I think about how I lost the following:

_____

_____

4. I try to numb myself when I think about how I lost the following:

_____

_____

5. One issue I feel I have completed grieving is the following:

_____

_____

6. I know that I still need to grieve more about

_____

_____

7. To help with my unexpressed grief I could

_____

_____

FOUR

PREVENTING AND
MANAGING RELAPSE

Relapse means the return of harmful feelings, thoughts, and behavior that were characteristic of us prior to beginning our dual recovery. We can relapse in our recovery from chemical dependency by taking mood-altering chemicals, thus endangering our safety and sobriety. We can relapse in our recovery from PTSD by engaging in unsafe behavior, such as allowing suicidal thinking or returning to an abusive relationship.

But we can also experience more subtle forms of relapse to PTSD. We can find that our old protector part once again kicks into full gear, causing us to be very critical of ourselves and others or to be very controlling. Or we may find that we are once again trying to do everything by ourselves, not asking anyone for help.

Making a distinction between a lapse and a relapse is helpful. We have a *lapse* when we briefly slip back into our old behavior but then quickly pull ourselves out of it and restart our recovery program. We have a *relapse* when we continue to engage in old patterns *and* do not use the new skills and support we have developed in our program to get ourselves back on track.

Recovery entails knowing ourselves well. We need to know not only which of our old behaviors are most likely to recur but also what might trigger a lapse or relapse.

The two main factors triggering a lapse to chemical use are (a) positive expectations of use and (b) managing negative emotions. *Positive expectation of use* refers to the thinking that life was or will be more enjoyable when drinking or using. People who glamorize the good old days, or who think that since they have worked on their PTSD, they can safely return to drinking and using, run the risk of relapse.

The antidote is to learn to enjoy life in recovery. Remember that we have so much to celebrate. We have been spared a fatal outcome from our illness of addiction. And we also can learn to laugh and play and feel good about ourselves in sobriety.

Managing negative emotions means using chemicals to self-medicate unpleasant feelings. If we start to believe that we can't take the pain without a drink or drug, we have fallen into a mode of thinking that increases the risk of a relapse. A good recovery program for PTSD and addiction can help us better deal with painful feelings through the social support found in Twelve Step meetings and through learning skills to safely cope with feelings.

Regardless of how well we work our program, we are likely to encounter situations and times when our recovery is at risk. The risk of relapse is part of recovery from any chronic illness, and we are in recovery from two illnesses. When a lapse occurs and a full-blown relapse is imminent (notice we say "when," not "if"), we need to have a relapse management plan to keep the lapse from becoming a relapse. We need to prepare ourselves for this possibility, much as we practice fire drills. Being prepared for a potential relapse, understanding our personal relapse triggers, and having a "fire drill" plan reduce the chance of relapse of either chemical use or old behaviors.

Relapse is *not* a sign that we have failed or that we are "bad." We must avoid being self-critical. It is simply a reminder that we are never done learning about ourselves, our diseases, and our recovery needs. If we should relapse, we best serve our recovery by taking it as a lesson about how powerful our diseases are. While in no way giving ourselves permission to continue in relapse, or minimizing the discouragement that a relapse can bring, we can see it as an opportunity to design an even better recovery program.

Remember, we are sick getting well, not bad getting good. We deserve to be treated with love and kindness by others and by ourselves. If friends, family members, or even our counselors get angry at us when we relapse, we have the right and responsibility to set a boundary with them and tell them that we deserve to be treated with love and kindness. If we are beating ourselves up, then we need to tell that not-so-helpful critical part of ourselves to back off. We need to ask ourselves, *Is it helpful to be so hard on myself?* We need to learn how to have love and compassion and forgiveness for ourselves, just like our Higher Power has for us.

The following exercise will help you identify triggers for relapse and pinpoint some things that you can do to prevent a relapse.

Recovery Activity: My Relapse Prevention Plan

1. I know that drinking or using is not an option for me today. The negative consequences of drinking or using include

_____
_____
_____

2. I sometimes think of hurting myself when

_____
_____
_____
_____

3. I drink and use to escape from

_____
_____
_____
_____

4. Some situations that trigger my desire to drink or use include

_____

_____

_____

5. Some people who trigger my desire to drink and use include

_____

_____

_____

This is because

_____

_____

_____

6. A person who triggers my desire to hurt myself or do something unsafe is

_____

_____

_____

7. A memory that triggers my wanting to hurt myself or do something unsafe is

_____

_____

_____

8. I feel like running away or even moving away when

_____

_____

_____

9. I feel like acting out sexually (or in some other unsafe way) when

_____

_____

_____

10. I no longer need to act out in these ways because

_____

_____

_____

11. (Skip this question if you are not on medication.) I want to stop taking my medication when

_____

_____

_____

12. Three fun activities I can do to replace drinking or using or hurting myself are

a. _____

_____

b. _____

_____

c. _____

_____

13. Three people I can call when I feel low or am thinking about relapse are

_____ phone number: _____

_____ phone number: _____

_____ phone number: _____

Recovery Activity: Recovering from Relapse

The purpose of this exercise is to help assure you that you can (a) pull out of a relapse and (b) use your relapse as an opportunity to strengthen your dual recovery program.

1. I relapsed because I

_____

_____

_____

2. The excuse I used was

_____

_____

_____

3. Before I relapsed, I could have prevented it by

_____

_____

_____

4. I did not honor my need for safety when I thought

_____

_____

_____

5. I might not have relapsed if I had

_____

_____

_____

6. One thing I learned about myself from my relapse is that

_____

_____

_____

7. Two things I am going to do differently to prevent a future relapse and stay safe are

a. _____

_____

_____

b. _____

_____

_____

8. Two reasons to forgive myself for relapsing and view it as a lesson, not a mistake, are

a. _____

_____

_____

b. _____

_____

_____

FIVE

FAITH AND FEAR

Hopelessness often accompanies a lifetime of constantly struggling to survive. Dealing day after day with the impact of serious trauma, while staying clean and sober, can be difficult at times.

We addicted survivors often feel that things are "never going to improve" and that we "will never be happy." When we are feeling down, we feel as if it may last forever. Yet when we are happy, we feel it is a temporary state. We have usually had a life riddled with losses. Not surprisingly, we may question the existence of a loving Higher Power. We may ask how a loving God could treat someone this way. But in recovery, we have hope and faith that if we work our program, things will work out as they are supposed to. Working a recovery program gives us a newfound freedom over our lives and the choices we make. Working the Steps is empowering to our recovery.

Also, we need to pay attention to our spiritual side. It's important to our recovery that we come to believe that *something* or *someone* can help us. Our ability to have hope and faith, and to continue to work a recovery program even during the tough times, relies on this foundation. Remember the slogan "This, too, shall pass."

Stop the pain and begin healing. It takes time; it takes effort. But recovery works. It's worth it. You're worth it.